The Path to Cultural Wellness

Seven Pillars of Recovery with Reflections and Meditations to Help Us Heal From the Effects of Bias

Sonia Bailey

Fire Forged Recovery

With love, honor, and respect for the Most High who gives us breath, and for the dear ones who have gone before us, having given all including their fight and their resistance, their hearts, and their lives.

For our future.

Foreword

Those who read this book are seriously in for a rewarding and revealing experience. Dada Sonia has been deliberate in every line and chapter of this wonderful compilation. The guidelines she has set in this work, *The Path to Cultural Wellness: Seven Pillars of Recovery to Help us Heal from the Effects of Bias*, are clear! It is simple and straightforward- implement what is instructed. If you want something as badly as you claim, you put in the intentional work for it, period. Anyone who truly wants to reclaim the scattered links to restoring their health and strength, as a descendant of Alkebu-Lan, will seek the necessary guidance to ensure that outcome. Descendants, particularly those of us who were physically dislodged from our Motherland, literally have this contributive awesomeness designed by Dada Sonia to use towards our reconciliation and healing. It's our responsibility now to get it done!

Mhi. A.K. Tosu

Jegna wa Alkebu-Lan

Introduction

Welcome to the Cultural Wellness Movement.

This is a collective journey away from all forms of associating ourselves— the descendants of Africa— with an identity that indicates we are lost, or that we ever were. We are not broken, nor victims, nor hopeless, nor less than anyone or anything. We were never slaves or chattel. True, someone made a calculated financial decision to feed us and themselves this propaganda hundreds of years ago, but these lies have nothing to do with our truth. That our ancestors were kidnapped— humans, trafficked— and enslaved, is the truth. With our innate strength and dignity, we are now called on to collectively get up out of the mire left behind by these events. Together, we hereby turn our backs and walk away from the carnage inflicted on us again and again since those times. As one, we claim our whole health and our right minds and we tolerate this madness no more.

I know what you might be thinking because it crossed my mind too. How dare we consider releasing our knowledge of the things that have happened to us? How can we turn our eyes away from all these horrible things that happened to our ancestors; to us? How can we consider doing this in an era where people who look like us are killed at the grocery store, just for wearing the skin? How can we let go of anything when, daily, another of us is needlessly killed, or dismissed, or fill-in-the-blank-here-about-to-day's-destruction-of-a-descendant-of-Africa? Add another fill-in-the-blank about today's insidious denial of an African descendant's talents or right to live, walk around freely, or have prosperity. Seriously, it is an everyday assault on our senses.

This journey is not created for— and does not address— the actions or lack of actions of people whose ancestors were not trafficked from Africa and enslaved throughout the world. It is true, we all need healing. This journey, however, is not that one— the one where the entire planet heals from these atrocities. As the saying goes, let's put on our own life jackets first, before we try to save anyone else.

Contents

Preparing for the Cleanse

This book is a 30-day detox. It is a cleanse. It is just like a series of actions you might take to reset your body if you had been, for example, eating in an unhealthy fashion, or taking a lot of medication.

You might do something like this if you were helping your body to heal from an illness. Medical providers routinely order a cleanse when they have to use imaging to look inside and see if anything is growing in our gut that should not be there. Whenever we need a 'reset,' or a process that allows us to 'take stock and find out what we need to get rid of so we can make room for a cure or a new version of ourselves, we start with a cleanse. Even if you have never undergone a cleanse, this description gives you an idea of what has to be done.

Most of us have never taken a cleanse quite like this one. These 30 days will guide us through a process of detoxifying our minds, bodies, and spirits from the effects of living with bias. Just to get through the day, we often take on thoughts, behaviors, or activities that do not make us feel good about ourselves. We may not even notice the changes. Needing to get on with our lives, to continue to meet the demands of work or school, family, or relationship, growing our empire, or whatever else is going on, we press on. If we are lucky, one day our body, mind, or spirit sends us an early notification: it is time to sit down and take a look within. The notification, maybe in the form of a headache, a stomachache, a bad mood, a sense of doom, or something else, lets us know that we need to change some factors before things get worse. If we have a daily or weekly routine that includes a process for self-care, we might heed this early warning and keep that appointment. More likely, because of the daily demands we have to meet, we just keep going. Then, the body, mind, or spirit has to send a more urgent notification, and then one after that, even more intense, and then another until it is the one we can no longer ignore: the serious physical, spiritual, or mental health concern or relationship problem. So why wait for that cranky call from the psyche? Take this cleanse now. Begin to free yourself from the effects of structural racism.

Now, this is not about external factors, like policy changes or reparations, or legal actions. This is about healing the parts of us that we do not talk much about. This is like a self-built infirmary and safe harbor that allows us to address unseen wounds. Expect a lot from beginning this process, yet do not expect 30 days to permanently address the needed repairs within us. There is no magic cure that will immediately disintegrate all of the horrible effects left over multiple generations or erase the daily stressors of living with bias. This is a way to put your feet on the road to full healing.

How to do it:

Spend a day reviewing the introduction and this preparation.

Spend four days on each Recovery Pillar:

Day one- Reflect on the Pillar and read the Chapter.

Day two- read the meditation preparing to complete it on the following day.

Day three- complete the meditation or reflection.

Day four- complete the activity.

When you have completed all four pillars, spend day 30 journaling about what you have experienced through the process and the parts of you most affected by it.

Here is what you should cover each week of the month:

Week 1:

Preparation for the Cleanse.

A Mental Oasis.

Pillar One.

Pillar Two.

Week 2:

Pillar Three.

Pillar Four.

Week 3:

Pillar Five.

Pillar Six.

Week 4:

Pillar Seven.

Reflection on your cleanse journey.

Write a summary of the things you will do next.

After the cleanse:

Take the cleanse again in three months. Notice what you have learned in the interim, and how you have changed.

Begin the process of reframing your existence. Release the hold that structural racism and the effects of bias have on you. Release those effects one cleanse at a time. Start here. Start now.

A Mental Oasis

I magine you have a beautiful productive tree in the yard where you live. The tree provides shade. It gives sustenance through the fruit it produces. It enriches the air you breathe. It enriches the soil within which it is planted. It enhances the beauty of the landscape for you and your neighbors. Just imagine all the gifts you get from the tree, and how wonderful you feel when you are near it. Revel in the knowledge that it will be there when you are gone for the day, and how it will still be standing there, majestic and useful when you come home day after day. Imagine that this tree is still there long after you have completed your journey on the planet and your heirs, or the next owners, have taken over. Think about how the new owners of the house enjoy this tree and the many gifts that it offers.

Like this tree, you are a part of the legacy of life. You provide sustenance, beauty, and immeasurable gifts to the community.

Now shift your focus to another kind of day with the tree. Someone else comes along and s/he says the tree makes the place too dark. The fruit attracts bugs and is not sweet or nutritious enough. The leaves are blowing all over and creating a mess and destroying the beauty of the neighborhood. The tree is absorbing too many resources because of the water it used from the community supply or the rainfall. Even the oxygen that the tree contributes is somehow tainted.

What would you do if you encountered this lunatic? After having so many lived years with the tree you know some truths about it. You would likely not engage with the lunatic at all.

Imagine yourself turning your gaze away and leaving the conversation. What would that be like? Imagine that the lunatic is left standing there alone, festering in his or her lies. What will s/he do with that bag of shame and lies now that you will not take it? What will they do since they were not able to unload the sick goods into your psyche? Really, who cares what they do with it? They haven't poisoned you. They haven't changed a single truth about the tree in your yard. Your tree is still beautiful, productive, life-sustaining, and enduring.

Using this metaphor, I hope you can see the value in turning your gaze away from claims of lunacy about your beauty. The time for listening to such foolishness is up. We only have time for truth and love. Your duty is to focus on the love within you. Make a daily practice of building your psychological strength for the journey ahead, the journey of recovery. Each day, identify the beauty and utility within you and people who look like you. Don't jump back into the pool of negativity.

Stop consuming the poisons given to you daily on your television or your radio, in your newspaper, in your social media feeds, and out of the mouths of people, including those who look like you but who are still ill because they don't yet have recovery. Stop eating the fruit. Do not consume hate and do not feed it to others. You have more important work to do.

Commit to start and end your healing journey grounded in love.

Chapter One

What does it mean to commit to start and end your healing journey grounded in love?

The first task is to commit to starting. During your life so far, hopefully, you have had the gift of committing yourself to a worthwhile task. You may have done this to meet a personal best goal, or to finish a project. A commitment of self involves resolving to do something despite obstacles that will come up. You should expect obstacles in this process, from within you and from outside.

The second task is to actually start. Carve out space in your life to immerse yourself in this process. You deserve 30 days of attention to this area of your life. By starting, you can assure that you are working towards an eventual end to the pain.

The third task is to recognize that this is a healing journey. The injuries you have acquired because of bias were not created overnight, and they will not be healed tomorrow. This is a rigorous journey, similar to training for an endurance event. The path to wellness requires participation from every aspect of you. If you want to be free of these problems, take the steps found in this tool.

The fourth task is to love. Decide now that you will begin this month-long process from a perspective of love: self-love, the love of the Force that created you, the love of those who lived and died before you that helped gain the freedoms that you have today. This is exactly the reason that we must avert our gaze from negativity. If our gaze remains locked on the daily crimes committed against us, we can see nothing else on the horizon of our minds besides those crimes. If we continue to consume these daily accounts of our victimization and death, we are constantly immersed in violence. There is no time left available to focus on the unbelievable beauty, talents, richness, potential, and truth that lives and thrives among us, and within you in particular. This is why we must begin our journey in love. We must commit to this process.

Turn away from any anger or hate, and focus on self-love, love of community, and love of those who laid down their lives for you throughout time.

Meditation on Self Love

What safe space have you created as your psyche's refuge? This refuge is a time, habit, or area where you go to heal from the daily wear and tear. If you don't have that space in your life, create it now, whether it is a physical environment like a room or an emotionally safe nook that you carry with you and enter regardless of whether you're alone or in a crowded room. You will use it throughout the book and ongoing.

Enter your safe space now. Make sure that you have a mirror with you for this meditation.

Sit or stand comfortably. Gaze into the mirror if you have sight. If you have no sight, experience the meditation with your hands or if you have no hands, use your mind's eye.   Drink in what it means to be a descendant of the Divine expressed through African heritage. Take your time, and starting at the top of your head, just notice what you see there. Regardless of the state of your head or your hair, appreciate it. Even if it is without hair, or if it is covered with someone else's hair right now, regard it with appreciation. Take in your natural head. Just appreciate it as it is, or as it might be without the use of hair extensions, weaved hair, or processing. Look at the beauty of it. If you can't see your natural head or your unprocessed hair readily, imagine it as if it was the last time you could see it. Look at, or if the hair is gone, notice how gorgeous you still are without it, or remember the beauty, even its wild resistance, and independent spirit, the tight curls, the texture. Experience the resistance to the evils of bias, the independence, and the twists and turns of which you are made.

Look at the hue of the skin. Is it ebony? Is it cocoa? Is it honey? What unique hue embraces you? Experience the smoothness, the warmth, the beauty of it. Have you noticed its timeless elasticity lately? This beautiful, public-facing organ deflects a lot of hostility from you every day. It absorbs and uses the beautiful light of the sun, and nutrients from the environment. It is curious, isn't it: how or why can an organ of its utility be despised simply for its color?

Look into your eyes, or remember them, or see them in your mind. Without any contacts or other adjustments, what color are they? Brown? Black? Are they blue? Are they green? Experience them as a part of the whole you. What has their color meant in your journey to claim your space in a culture that has not welcomed the skin that surrounds them?

Regard with gratitude the strength and utility of your arms and legs, hands and feet, even your torso. These are your suit of armor in your role as a warrior in this war you never asked for.

Think about any depictions you have seen that frame your natural appearance as not being beautiful, as needing to be something else. Release those depictions with love. Release those other concepts of 'normal' as not belonging to you. Commit to identifying any ways you have allowed those ideas to seep into your consciousness.

Consider your wisdom, talents, and strengths. Do you disparage and deny them daily? Review them now. Think about your intellect, regardless of the extent of your formal training. Give thanks for the many days and ways that you have been guided through perilous or happy times. Vow to recognize these aspects of yourself daily.

Take a few deep breaths and consider the times that you have felt ashamed of your African ancestry. Have you regarded yourself as separate and distant from 'those people' who, you are told, descend from poverty and ignorance, who are savage in action or appearance, who try to keep each other down, who are lazy and shiftless? Vow to explore daily how these beliefs are put forward to perpetuate oppression. In your safe space, dismiss these lies and embrace the truths. Commit to learning more about the wealth, talents, skills, and brilliance embodied in you and people who share your ancestry and current experience.

Once you have accepted and loved yourself without any changes, have a new experience of yourself, grounded in self-love. After you have undergone this cleanse to remove from yourself any ideas that the way that you are is flawed and that you need 'enhancements' to be acceptable, it may be safe to go back to using whatever fashions you feel help you to best express yourself and highlight your strengths. Keep in mind that 'enhancements' are usually things we add to make ourselves more likely to fit in with European culture. Nothing that you can add to your body, however, can erase or minimize your African ancestry.

Use this exercise as often as needed to remove from yourself any ideas that your natural and beautiful appearance is flawed. Begin each day with a five-minute reflection during which you practice loving who and what you are just as you were created.

Activity- Love in Community

Go to a mall, barber or beauty shop, park, or another place where you can find a flow of African descendants. As an alternative, and only if you can't get out of your living situation, try using television programming or a movie.

Take a seat in a comfortable spot where you can observe. Find the darkest, then the lightest person in the environment who appears to be of African descent. Notice and release any judgments that spring to your mind immediately about the person(s). If you didn't like the way they were dressed, how they carried themselves, or what they were doing, let go of these observations. File them away so you can think more about them later, as you may find more information about the biases you carry about yourself or others. But for now, focus on the beauty you observe in them. You will recognize these more easily, having just found them in yourself. See the rich hues, the resilience, the air of timeless regalness. Imagine their journey starting with their ancestors and thinking forward to today, to their children or grandchildren, or great-grandchildren, while they have been wearing that skin. Imagine what strengths and weaknesses they must have expressed. Think about the ways they expressed resistance to discrimination and bias, and the times they believed they failed to resist. See all of the ways that their journey might have echoed your own. Embrace it all.

Educate Yourself. Acknowledge the Truth of History.

Chapter Two

In the current era, there's a lot of conversation in America about our history not being spoken about because: 'it brings up pain for black people,' or 'it hurts white people's feelings,' or 'slavery is over, just move on.' Whatever color their skin is, some people roll their eyes when topics around racial healing are raised. Truly, people are just done with talking or thinking about this and wish in vain that there was some 'get it over with once and for all' button that we could push so that these conversations and their causes would be resolved. Wouldn't that be great? Maybe.

The truth is that we must look at it, deeply. We must know exactly what happened and how we got here. This is the only path to healing— to understand. We need to know the pain of our history and we need to know more about where we come from. This is a time to explore and learn about what we lost.

What were the values, beliefs, norms, ceremonies, and rituals, that belonged to Africa? Which traditions were carried forward? What effect do those traditions have on us today?

If you ask the garden-variety descendant of the continent of Africa anything about African history before the transatlantic trading of kidnapped people, you'll find that many are plagued with hurt, shame, and feelings of abandonment because the one thing we have been told is this: that our own people sold us into slavery. The very narrative around slavery blames us for our condition. Intergenerational trauma means that we feel the impact of this betrayal as if we experienced it as intimately as our ancestors did. We have shame about the perpetuated ideas that surround us about our origins; that Africa is materially and spiritually impoverished and worthless; that Africans hate American 'Blacks'; that we are a country-less people with no real origins and no roots. Africa is not ours to claim, the lies say.

We need to learn about where it all began, centuries and centuries before the transatlantic human trafficking trade. For thousands of years, we governed ourselves through systematic means. We had kindness and conflict. We had order and chaos, values and immorality, chastity & cheating, love & hate, marriage & divorce, family & solitude, jobs & unemployment, birth & death. If we look more honestly at history and go beyond that which is available even in history textbooks not researched or authored by people of Africa, we'll continue to believe that we traded or sold each other, enslaved others, or became enslaved. But do you know what really happened? The human trafficking was started even before the Europeans joined in almost 900 years later, although this information isn't commonly available or discussed. We need to look closely at the things we have accepted as being truth. We know for sure that we experienced unspeakable horrors that our ancestors could not have understood, having never seen or experienced them, but there is much more that we need to know.

Slavery and war, regardless of who incites or perpetuates them, are horrors. A key difference in our story was the kidnapping and human trafficking, which resulted in a particularly brutal kind of imprisonment. We were regarded as property, and deep lies and structures were built and perpetuated in our realities and our minds to try to contain us. We were treated with unspeakable cruelty. Our attempts to rebel or escape were often met with death, dismemberment, and other horrors. These cruelties were not personal, just necessary so that the human traffickers could maintain themselves at the apex of power. Yet, we were not contained. We enacted resistance at every turn, and we still enact resistance to structural racism today.

Our job now is to educate ourselves and generations to come about these truths and every other truth about our ancestry, the rich traditions and, history that gave us life, and the strengths from this system that are still alive in our DNA. [1] To prevent this exploitation of our resources and our kidnapping and enslavement from ever happening again, we must know it personally. We must vow never to forget.

We must also get up. We must rise from the myths and realities of our disempowerment. By summoning our strength to squarely face the truth, we strengthen ourselves for the tasks of recovery.

It is almost impossible to educate ourselves by listening exclusively to people who do not share our ancestry, or by heeding popular television, radio, movies, podcasts, social media feeds, or even family and friends who have not bothered to educate themselves. We can —- we must—-teach ourselves to fact-check everything we read, see, hear or experience. Get curious about what happened, and how the past influences your life today. Become a 'lay researcher'- a person who explores

---

1. https://medlineplus.gov/genetics/understanding/basics/dna/

parts of life from a perspective of learning. Take a class, or develop and teach one for your community. You are fully equipped to educate yourself and your household as you find credible sources of information and begin to discern repeating patterns that guide you to the truth.

Meditation on Knowing

What would it be like if you could speak with someone from the past? Time travel may be real someday, but for now, we don't have it as a tool, so we have to devise other ways of knowing about the past so that we can embrace it, be free of its pain, and stand firm in who we are today.

What questions would you ask if you could find that single person who could give insight into our present-day condition? For example, why were we trafficked and imprisoned, then treated like a scourge for the next four hundred years? What makes us different from other groups of people who have been subject to a cataclysm (defined as a sudden, violent upheaval, especially in a political or social context)? How can we extinguish all forms of oppression directed at us today? How can we seize our minds and our attention away from any initiatives that detract from our full freedom and self-control? Answers exist to all of these and other questions. You can know this information. Knowing will require that you change your point of view. With this 30-day cleanse, you must release any expectation that the system which benefits from your imprisonment in your habits and your mind will help you find a way out. But you are strong and intelligent. Get up now and walk towards liberty.

Knowledge Activity

Write down ten questions about your African heritage and history that you want the answer to. Carve out a dedicated time in your day when you can again use your safe space. During this time, as you read each question, explore the knowledge base you have built within. Explore other ways that you find answers. Do you use prayer? Reading? Self-reflection? The wisdom of a knowledgeable group? Walking or running? Your reasoning skills? Explore these resources to begin to identify the answers to your questions. Jot down the answers and observations. Us the internet, a research library, bookstores, and local legends to get more information about what you want to know. Reflect on the findings, a little each day and more fully every time you take this 30-day cleanse. Continue your research as you move through the days and years ahead.

Actively grieve things that were taken, and things that you've lost. Mourn with others who've shared the journey.

Chapter Three

W hat is the cost of unresolved grief? Most experts on grief will tell you that people who don't deal with a loss end up with serious effects, like withdrawal from everyday activities, detachment from family, or lack of trust in other people. Other, potentially even more serious effects include depression, low self-esteem, and unhealthy attachments to substances, behaviors, or activities. People with unresolved grief may act as if nothing happened or become obsessed with the loss on the opposite end. Sometimes we get into legal trouble. Does any of this sound familiar? Most of us know at least one person of African descent that displays one or more of the above behaviors. No matter how many times someone tells us to 'just get over it', full wellness can elude us until we face this.

Have you considered the grief that you may have as a descendant of Africa? Our casualties have been unimaginable. When you consider the losses of place, people, identity, potential, and wealth that we have inherited over the generations because we have not resolved these issues, the healing journey may seem daunting. Add to our historical load the events of the present day— the continuous crimes against us as we stubbornly persist in wearing this skin (as if we would shed it even if we could), the daily news of our demise, the lack— and recovery seems impossible.

Recovery and wellness are fully possible for us. We must heal now, for ourselves, and on behalf of our youth and the generations to come. We can start by acknowledging the truth that collectively, we have few opportunities to embrace a natural, healing, and cleansing process of grief. We can then create these opportunities.

Much has been written, and a lot of information is available, about the effects of grief, and experts have begun to write about the particular grief of African descendants. Acknowledge the losses. Educate yourself about how to heal from losses and traumatic events. Give yourself the needed support to change by embracing this process. Contact a grief support expert of African descent if you find that you can't get through it alone.

Participate in at least one personal, and one group memorial service that formally acknowledges your release from any attachment to the Atlantic Human Trafficking Trade. Such a ceremony helps us turn our backs and walk away from our identity being held hostage by those events. Sharing the experience of grieving about these losses with other people who have the same history offers healing that we cannot achieve in any other way.

Follow the release with a celebration of your new life, free of these psychological chains.

Meditation on Mourning

By now you are used to using your safe space. Enter it now to prepare for a thorough self-examination of your grief related to your history.

Consider ways that unresolved grief related to being a descendant of Africa torn away from norms, traditions, and identity has affected you. Reflect on this: how might your life have been better or different if the generations before you had been raised with full identity and history intact? What if you knew exactly who your ancestors were for the last twenty generations? Suppose wealth accumulated in those generations had now become yours to safeguard, expend, and grow for those next born? This passing down of resources used to be referred to as 'coming from old money.' As descendants of Africa, most of us have not had the privileges that this continuity of access and supply would have offered. Instead, we have needed to create our own success alone. The desire to make our mark or find a moment of ease gained by our individual accomplishments has separated us from our sense of collective responsibility and growth. We may believe that we must succeed alone or be 'dragged down' by people who look like us but have not achieved sufficient success on their own.

What talents might have been cultivated and refined, century after century, until they now bloomed, fully mature, in you? What if the formulas, cures, equations, and recipes, had been handed down to you intact, instead of your having to research them and piece them back together as best you could? Imagine how these same dynamics affected relationships, national allegiances, business development, education, health, and joy. These are among the things taken or lost by the trafficking, imprisonment, and abuse of our ancestors.

Write or record a statement of things you have lost due to the effects of bias. Acknowledge how those things have hurt you.

What aspects of this pain would you like to be released from? Consider the areas of your life that will change for the better when you have found this freedom.

Mourning Activity

On August 20, 2022, at the shores of the Atlantic Ocean, the same ocean the first of us crossed when we were trafficked to this continent, a group gathered for a Requiem for Slavery. This first annual event was a marker of the official day that we symbolically returned this atrocity to the depths from which it arose. Together, we committed to lay down any ties we had to consuming the toxins so readily offered to us every day— words, gestures, or anything else suggesting we were inferior or broken.

Create such a ceremony for yourself now. Use the list you created in the meditative activity as a base. Design a reading, song, or poem that represents what you are letting go of. Add relevant drumming or music. You can even add a dance or a dramatic performance that reflects the release and celebration.

Use some physical expression representing your release. Say a prayer, release sand, pour water, or ceremonially burn pieces of paper upon which you have written the things that you are releasing.

Invite loved ones to participate with you. Help them prepare for the release event, then schedule a day and time when you can complete it together. Tell your friends and community about the release. Include others who wish to join you.

Send a photo or one-minute video of your ceremony to us at TheCultureCures@fireforgedrecovery.com. We'll archive these events to show current and future generations our stories of healing.

Release Hate Directed Inward and Outward.

Chapter Four

Have you ever heard the old saying, "Holding on to anger is like drinking poison and expecting the other person to die?" That's not a good strategy, but it is what we do when we refuse to look at how angry we are about our experiences of racism in this society. Hate, described as intense or passionate dislike, is the result of our anger. We direct that hate at ourselves and we harbor it towards others.

Let's put the poison down.

Even those of us who function very well can be filled with anger. In daily life, hundreds of actions or events encourage us to direct anger inward. Without our even noticing, this insidious anger could be infecting our thoughts and emotions because of the overbearing yet unseen influence of structural racism:

-anger over our failure to be 'white', or our failure to be acceptable to 'white society.' That is, our failure to transmute our skin, our heritage, and our essence into something more acceptable to the European ethos.

This may lead us to find subtle ways to 'get inside' or gain access to the places where all those resources are: wherever 'white' people are. We begin to disparage other African descendants, dismissing them because they have the same problems we do and they can't help us get anywhere.

-anger and self-hate about the alternating thoughts and feelings within us; African pride one moment, and in the next moment, that compelling desire to join 'them' and be acknowledged and accepted.

-anger about failure to stop doing whatever it is we are apparently doing wrong, which results in our not getting the resources or respect we work so hard for.

We don't talk about this very much because it is so unpleasant to face. We can be free of these mental challenges. Imagine how fabulous that freedom is going to feel.

To be completely free of hate, we must also acknowledge the anger that we have towards people with non-African skin. This anger and hatred are triggered afresh every time we hear another story on the news or experience another slight in the store where someone overlooks us in line. What about when we're with a 'white-skinned' friend or coworker at a restaurant or other setting, and we notice how the person serving us will look that person in the eye or talk to that person without even acknowledging that we're there? This scenario plays out over and over, day after day, encompassing our whole being. We never quite know whether it's our skin alone, or our skin and gender, our skin and our education level, our skin and our income level, our skin and the way we worship, our skin and the way we dress, but we know for sure that the skin is a factor.

Remember that none of these reactions have anything to do with you. These actions by people with the other skin result from the flip side of the same virus that we are cleansing ourselves of. It's the racial equivalent of a zombie virus. There is no actual inferiority in you. Release bring controlled by the anger, the shame, and the pain that rises in you every time someone treats you as if their fantasy of you as an inferior being is real. Release the ways you have allowed these reactions to affect how you feel about yourself and your fellow descendants of Africa. We must channel the anger into productive use as we cure ourselves from this terrible condition.

How are we directing that anger and hate at our brothers and sisters? Do we disparage them in our daily speech? Do we encourage them to internalize and carry the anger and hate toward people with the other skin? Do we carry every negative story and regurgitate it to them? Do we encourage them to alter their actions or appearance, away from things associated with African heritage in favor of things more acceptable in Euro culture? Maybe we deny their experiences of racist treatment and tell them to 'just get over it.' Examine yourself for signs of internalized resentment over lost self-worth that you inflict on our beloved ones. Discontinue these actions immediately.

Meditation on Releasing Hate

F ind your well-used and comfortable safe space. Relax within it, and notice how safe you feel in this environment that you've created.

Think about the last five racist episodes that you've seen or heard about in the last year. Did they happen at a nearby grocery store, office, park, or restaurant, in a loved one's tale, or a news story?

Imagine that you have a special device that allows you to see physical symptoms of the racism virus. In your mind's eye, reexamine those five episodes while using this device. Practice seeing the reality that the virus causes irrational behaviors in the people who have it. Feel comfortable in the knowledge that none of the symptoms displayed by the infected people have anything to do with reality. Also notice that the virus makes the infected dangerous, just like the fictionalized zombies.

Fortify yourself with the knowledge that people affected by this virus say and do things to harm you because they are in an altered reality that is not based on truth. Release hate towards yourself, your community, and the infected.

Activity- Releasing Hate

Now that you have mastered seeing skin color-based hate as a disease, take your observations live. Just as you did before, go to a place where you'll encounter many African descendants and others. A mall in an upscale area might offer you a great opportunity for observation.

Find a seat where you can people-watch uninterrupted, or if you feel up to it, walk around. This time, use your 'virus lens' perspective. Notice any looks or interactions that come in your direction, whether welcoming or disparaging. What is remarkable about these interactions? Are people eyeing you as if they regard you as an equal, or do you sense condescension? Do people of African descent avoid you or make eye contact? With your new dedication to releasing hate, how do you find yourself reacting to people's responses to you?

Jot down notes for yourself if you find things that you can study later, which will help you to heal. If difficult reactions arise, practice releasing them as if doing so protects your health. It does.

Continue to observe, using your mental 'virus lens.' At the end of the day, share your observations with someone you trust.

Begin to Heal From the Inside Out. Commit to Healing More Every Day.

Chapter Five

This pillar can be a tough one because asking people of African descent to open up, then look at, or heaven forbid tell someone about, struggles that we are having, is a bit taboo. For centuries, opening up and talking about our issues was dangerous, even life-threatening if the information got into the wrong hands. After all, in the Northern Hemisphere and around the world, we gained freedom from imprisonment through underground means which required the ability to keep a secret. But this is a new day, and we need to clean out some closets.

We are making progress in this area. Many of us are using tools like therapy, counseling, coaching, and mentoring as tools to help us heal from the inside. The catalyst is often that we want to express our whole selves and rich talents to our community and the world. To do that, we have to let someone see who we are, and allow them to help us hone our skills.

There are other methods of healing from the inside out, many of which do not involve talking with someone else. Your healing is of primary importance. Regard all paths to healing as valid and useful, and select the one that works for you. Just remember that talking with someone who can help is an excellent tool.

Selecting well is the key. Choose someone who knows what you face wearing the skin as you walk around this society. Ask questions before you make your selection. Make sure their focus matches yours, and avoid choosing someone because they are popular, or because they charge the most or the least.

Another reason that healing from inside is difficult is that recovery involves taking responsibility for personal behavior and doing some work to get rid of habits that don't serve you. Recovery involves looking at every self-sabotaging behavior, every way that we silently grieve, every issue that we medicate with measures such as sex, money, shopping, overspending, drugs, religion, movies, food and more.

This calls for reexamining our relationship with everything. What do you do when you're in pain about anything? Do you know the root causes of your pain, and what the origin is? What is disintegrating you from the inside? Do you drill down to that core issue every time you've floundered and used a poor coping tool?

This is what you have to do at the bottom of every bucket of ice cream or that last slice of cake, maxed out credit card, or when you wake up on yet another morning with that sexual partner who it's always a bad idea to interact with, and so on.

Don't worry if you can't change these behaviors the very first time you try. Commit to healing more every day. Ask for help.

Meditation on Healing

By now you know where to go for these meditations: the safe space you have carved out for this. Be there now.

Relax and reflect on your last disappointment, your last bad day, your last injury from racism. Think about the last conflict you had with a loved one that didn't end well, or with which you are not satisfied with how you coped. What did you use to manage your feelings? What is something healthier that you could have turned to instead? Decide which healthier coping and release mechanism you'll use the next time you reach a difficult crossroad.

Healing Activity

What area in need of healing will you commit to begin to work on today? Pick only one concern at a time, and work through it until it is healed before you take on the next one.

What system of accountability will you set up for yourself to help you get it done? A system of accountability is a series of checks and balances that you put in place so that when you don't want to meet the goal you set, someone is going to ask you about it. Whether that's telling a (healthy, trustworthy) friend, telling a coach, telling a therapist, or telling your mother, sister, or brother what the plan is, someone has to know. You also need to train your partner in accountability about what you want them to say when you give them that lame excuse about why you didn't accomplish your step. For this part, you may want to select a coach, since helping you tolerate the intolerable in yourself will not be a possible outcome. Whoever you choose, make sure they understand the journey upon which you are asking them to support you.

The first time you do this activity, your concerns about putting your business in the street or being thought of as 'less than' or 'broken' may flare up. Counter these concerns by choosing someone who will keep your confidence and who you trust in other ways. Make sure the person you ask for help has the time and emotional space to assist you, especially if you select family or a friend. If you begin to feel too stressed out or too sad, get more formal support.

Find and Stay Focused On Your True and Immeasurable Worth.

Chapter Six

A conversation about our true and immeasurable worth is hard to find in society, especially for people of African descent. Many forums reinforce lies about our valuelessness. This valuelessness seems to have been created during our imprisonment, when we were referred to as property. A lot of energy was put into building that concept in us and everyone else. This was true not only in the Northern Hemisphere but around the world; that we were a subspecies, so to speak. We were said to be less than everything else; almost inhuman. Almost animal-like. Even though we have come many years away from the origins of these insane ideas, the institution of bias and its effects still rages rampant in today's world.

How do you define your worth? What do you think makes you valuable? Regardless of your belief system, it is evident that some intelligence, power, or spirit greater than us created us and that Force endowed us with certain properties that give us mastery over the earth if we can take it. If you start with the concept of your creation and move forward, you can begin to see your magnificence. Your ability to do the things that other species on this planet can't do is evidence to your greatness. If you layer on top of that all of the things that happened before this day to make your existence possible, you can further illustrate the value of your magnificence and your greatness in the grand scheme of things.

As a person of African descent, think about the more than two thousand years that passed before you were born. Think about that even though the earth is billions of years old, Africa is well documented as the seat of civilization; the seed of creation. So if life started there and spread out elsewhere, just think about the history, power, and greatness embedded in your DNA. Walking yourself forward from that reality gives you a basis for finding your greatness. Whatever trials and tribulations your life contains today are temporary circumstances. Even seemingly intractable conditions like poverty, lack of access to resources, and lack of ability to surmount the problems of systemic racism alone or as a group can be temporary. Don't be daunted by these difficulties. Find this greatness not only from your ancestry and creation but from who you are today as a person who thrives despite difficult circumstances and odds that seem unbeatable.

The people who rely on you for help are waiting for you to see yourself as they see you, so they can benefit from the gifts of your being.

Activity- The Worth Party

W hat you'll need: a nice room or park, a microphone, paper, pens, a surface to write on,
sparkling cider or water, chairs, and nice glasses Host
a Worth Party in your community.

Invite people, and ask them to come dressed in fine
garments that reflect their internal value. When they
arrive, they are now titled Notables. Ask each Notable
to write their one-paragraph biographical statement,
which includes their awesomeness as they would like
a room full of people to hear it when they are intro-
duced.

Ask the group to sit in one or more circles. Ask each
Notable to pass their finished bio to the person on their
right. The person who receives the bio must add one
sentence of something wonderful about the Notable,
then pass that bio to their right. Keep passing the bios
to the right until every Notable has his or her bio back.

When every Notable has his or her bio back, they should pass it to the person on their left, who will read it aloud. Act as the Master of Ceremonies to welcome each speaker as they introduce each Notable, using the microphone to read the bio. All listeners should provide a standing ovation for each Notable.

At the end of the party, each Notable should write and recite a personal oath to find and stay focused on his or her true and immeasurable worth. The group should set a date for the next Worth Party, where they will hold accountability for each Notable by finding out how they have fulfilled this oath during the time since the prior Worth Party.

Help Your Community Live Its Potential.

Chapter Seven

N one of us lives in a vacuum, even though we feel so alone. This feeling of aloneness is a part of our human condition. Even twins, sometimes identical twins, feel that they're alone. Twins may have the advantage of feeling a little more connected to another person, but they too feel the separation of their experience, even though you can't get closer to another human than sharing a womb with them. After the womb, however, they too have to walk their own path. The rest of us swiftly and closely encounter the bitter reality that we came into this world alone and we'll leave it alone, regardless of our intimate connections. Daily we battle this sense of aloneness and figure our way through this landscape. Some of us are fortunate to have partners who share a lifetime and rich experiences with us. Others of us are fortunate to have lifelong connections with family or solid friends, through thick and thin. Despite these close connections, we still struggle in our darkest moments to feel that connectedness.

Recovery and wellness help us to identify that we are not alone. We are always immersed in something deeper than ourselves, something that we can rely on for strength, regardless of our faith system. Spiritual beliefs offer guidance and a moral compass that point us to the Divine, which gives us strength and support.

There are, however, several significant ways that we are connected with others. Good or bad, we're connected with our communities, our families, friends and associates, colleagues and coworkers, our neighborhoods, states, our country, and our world. As descendants of Africa, we have a world community of people who look like us and with whom we share DNA, and who literally are experiencing many of the same conditions we face daily, regardless of where they are in the world. They may speak any language. Our shared experience lies in how we are regarded because of our skin. The impacts of our imprisonment affected every continent and many places in the world where people of African descent live.

When the trafficking ships started running, they dropped us off at the highest bidder. Regardless of where we came from, if the skin looked like ours, we were treated in the same way. The traffickers gave no preferences.

You can see that the job of helping our community live its potential has many levels. Our responsibility begins with ourselves. We must live our potential before we can help our descendants, our children, and our larger community of friends or family or neighborhood to live theirs.

This is our duty and responsibility: to collectively help each other live our potential, whether it is locally, nationally, or globally. Because we all share this experience of needing to find wellness after the traumatic events that happened to us four hundred years ago, we share the imperative to get ourselves and our collective consciousness out of the current and residual insanity. We cannot allow it to continue anymore.

Can you imagine what life will be like when we have done this? Envision our new narrative, where we internalize our true and immeasurable worth daily instead of swallowing the bitter daily doses of the latest tragedies that we endure.

Meditation on Immeasurable Worth

L ook closely at your daily life. Can you truly say that you are intimate with your greatness and that you express it every day starting when your feet hit the floor first thing in the morning? If this is not true of you today, write down three ways that you'll begin to make it true.

Develop a mechanism to remind yourself daily to use your abilities to improve your life and someone else's. of this greatness of your capacity, your history, and your capabilities. Each day, use this mechanism to help yourself grow fully into all of who you are. Never again evaluate your worth according to someone else's definition.

Activity- Community Potential

A mong us lie the solutions to the current problems we face as descendants of Africa. We have the ideas and strategies that will allow us to better our world and achieve wellness and freedom from the effects of bias. The culture has the cure. We are the culture. Let's hold ourselves and the community to high standards in principle and practice as we care for each other.

Let's find and cultivate the many talents and experts among us, applying these gifts to our development. Here are two ways you can start:

Host a meeting for your immediate family and closest friends. Talk about what keeps each of you from living to your highest potential. Explore the reasons presented to identify any ways in which these limitations have been made worse by unresolved barriers resulting from bias. Develop a list of priorities that will help each person rise above these limitations and begin the tasks of healing. Make a plan to follow through on the group's suggestions. Set a date when you will come back together to measure progress.

Research and develop an African history workshop for your family and friends. Host this workshop within three months of developing it. Incorporate ongoing African history workshops into family gatherings.

Reflection on Community

We have been fractured by the ways we've been torn apart over time. We have been separated from kin and nations by human traffickers and circumstances. Let's rebuild our connections locally, nationally, and globally. The most difficult part of this work begins in our homes.

Spend a day with loved ones. Regard your actions towards them. How often do you talk with the people you live with about the effects of bias? Do you perpetuate bias in your home or family, perhaps by favoring loved ones who have more European physical characteristics like lighter skin or straighter hair? Are your private conversations laced with African-hating language, where you deny your heritage or encourage others to deny theirs? Do the goals you hold for your children encourage them to adopt European values and measures of success, without regard for their African heritage?

Closely examine what you encourage loved ones to do, and the language you use in speaking with them. Do you use words that others use to disparage people of African descent, and then make excuses about why these terms are acceptable coming from you?

How can you strengthen the community where you live?

Take a walk or a ride around your neighborhood. Look around.

In your opinion from this superficial observation, has every person you see lived up to his or her potential? Why or why not? Do you think each person would see his or her value the same way you see it?

What support do we need from each other to live this potential? How will you help your community to see the talent and beauty within? What will you do personally to help people raise their awareness about the fact that we need to get rid of this virus that keeps us stuck in brokenness? Write your ideas down. Share them with a few members of your family and your community and make a plan to act on them.

We've only begun

Our healing is a serious matter. Applaud yourself for beginning your detoxification from this virus. Remember that you are the living, breathing cure for this ailment. Only we can change the outcomes that we have been experiencing.

Have confidence in the knowledge that as each of us becomes healthy, we will soon develop a critical mass—a point where more of us have found cultural wellness than the number of us who have not. This critical mass will begin to make the needed changes even as the others are merely starting on their journey. Rise to your role as an architect of our recovery and wellness.

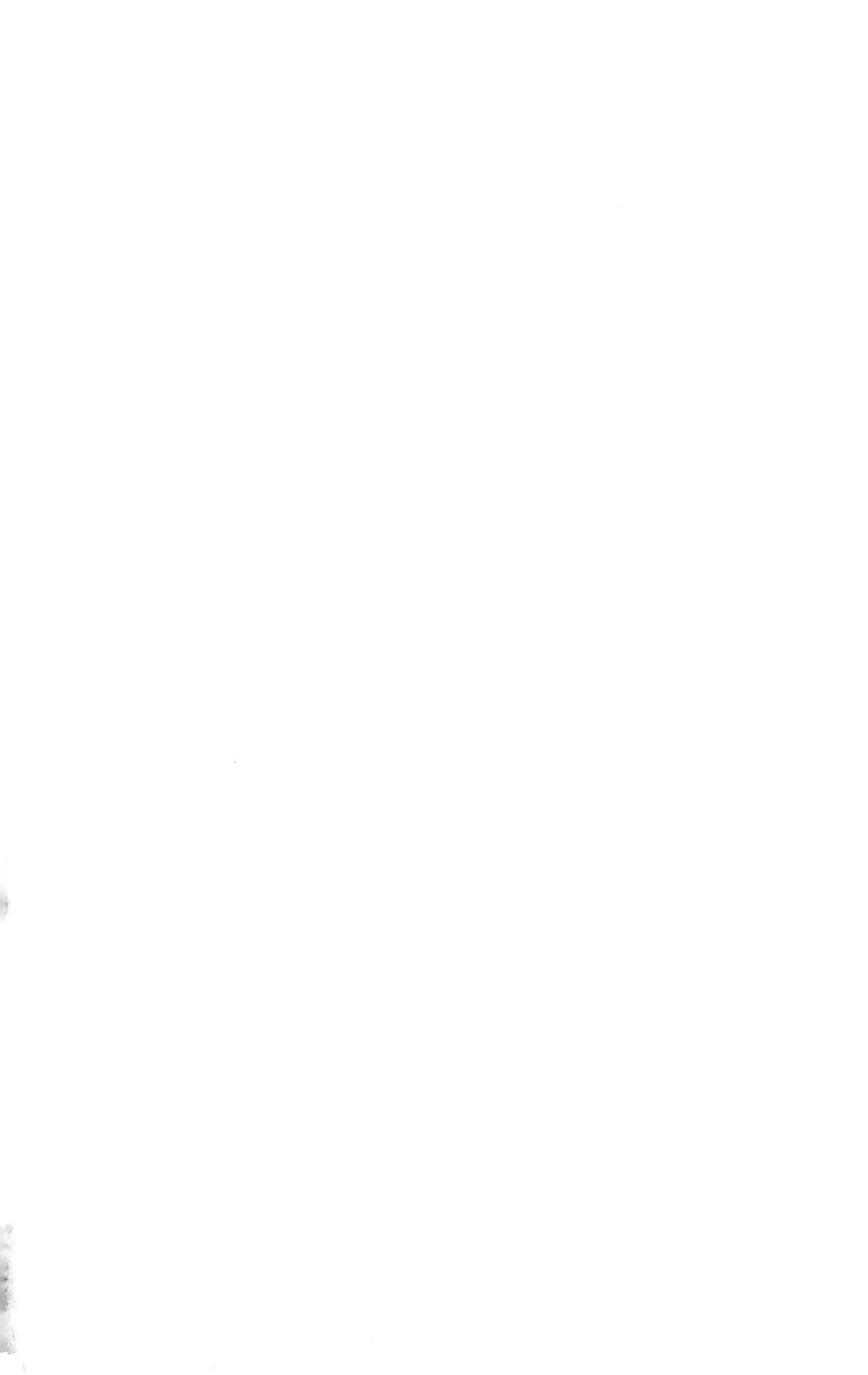